HEY

FATTY

FATTY!

Because SOMEONE needs to smack you in the head.

A Body Fat Management Manual

By: Craig Charles Bauer

Fat Management Instructions:

Step #1   Read This Entire Manual First!

Step #2   EXERCISE By Following YOUR HEART!

Step #3   WAIT UNTIL YOU ARE HUNGRY To Eat Food!

Step #4   EAT FOOD Until You Are Not Hungry!

Step #5   RELAX And Adapt.

Step #6   Repeat Steps 2 – 5 for the rest of your life!

YES! It is THAT easy.

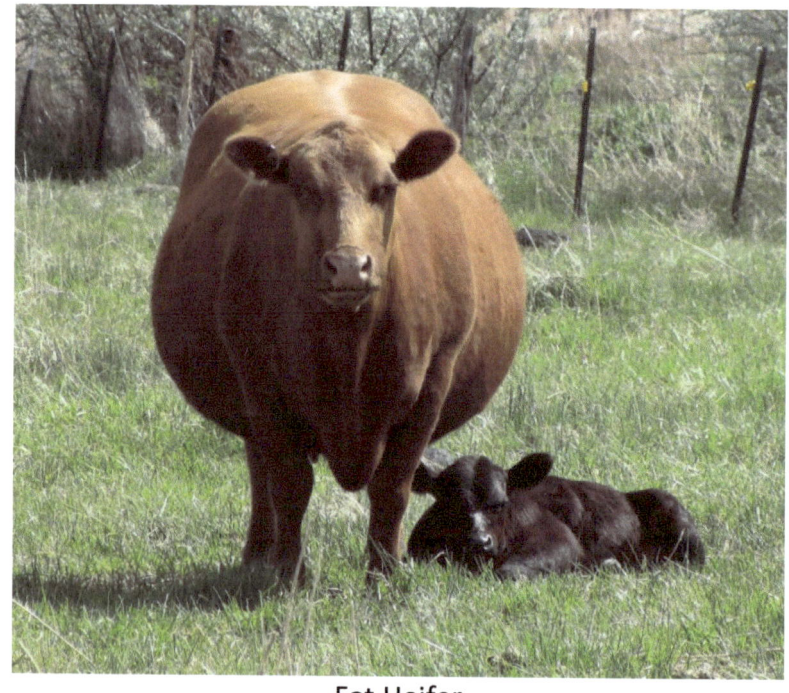

Fat Heifer

Because people like to sue

DISCLAIMER: All actions taken by individuals who read and/ or use the information presented herein are taking action(s) of their sole volition, discretion, decision and of their own free will. The author and/or his representatives, successors and/or heirs assume no liability for action(s) taken either directly or indirectly as a result of reading or learning of the material contained herein regardless of how this informational material was acquired by the user. All actions taken by individuals as a result of this Informational material are taken solely of their own conscious thought and conscious directive decision. This Manual is not intended as a substitute for Clinical Medicine or Prescription Drug treatment and does NOT take into consideration all possible medical conditions or other In-competences. All individuals, entities and/or groups, whether natural or not, assume all liability for the usage of the material herein and assume all risks associated with the actions and ideas forwarded by these writings. The Author Presents this work as an original work of Informational Art and any and all similarities to other productions, reproductions, persons, writings, or other resources of any kind is purely coincidental.

*Seek the guidance of a medical professional before starting a diet and exercise routine especially if you are pregnant or have existing health concerns.

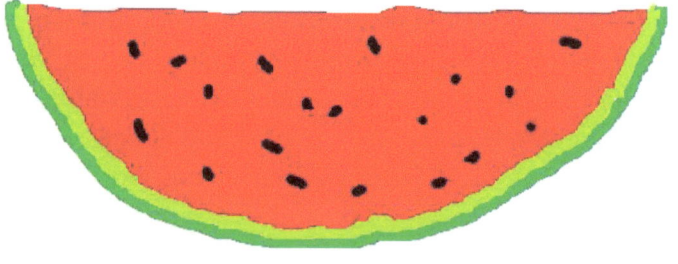

This manual is based upon the observation and study of life and living factors here on planet earth. It is designed as a simplified manner in which to re-establish your natural tendency to regulate your metabolism beneficially.

Ultimately it is up to YOU to regulate body fat. No one else will, or even CAN, do this for you.

EXERCISE by following YOUR HEART!

Exercise is one of them nasty words. Well, DO IT ANYWAY. Do something! Exercise doesn't have to be a workout at the gym, where people gawk at your gut peeking out from beneath your tee shirt, and it certainly doesn't mean competition. It simply means getting your Body in motion. MOVE! Got pains and aches, well so does everybody else. Wanting PITY because your feet are sore is not going to make that big, old, huge, ASS melt away! Moving that large loaded butt around will make it smaller and delightfully, many of your aches and pains will disappear along with blobs of UN-NECESSARY FAT.

Link: Many ailments are simply caused by inactivity and poor blood/fluid circulation.

Workouts do not need to be extreme aerobics, weight lifting, or a battle of Ninja Masters. How about Shopping at the mall? Golfing? Walking the dog? Your four legged pal is a VERY good comparison to judge fitness levels from. Let's DEFINITELY mention the bonus of taking that loud, barking, fur ball for a stroll and ENCOURAGING him to Pee on everything in the neighborhood. Wasn't that better than watching him pee on things inside your home?

Link: Calories burned walking the dog.

Here's a short list of exercises that aren't exercise:

Auto Repair. Put a 1200 horse power Big Block in your Toyota or something.

Horse Shoeing. This is a skill anyone can learn and it's difficult.

Goat ropin'. Gotta goat? Gotta Rope? Go for it!

Hang gliding. Can't beat the feeling of FLYING as a form of exercise.

Roller blading. Ok, so it's a sport. SO WHAT!

Wandering Around a City. Do it aimlessly for maximum purpose-free exercise. (No, not in a car.)

Dancing. Whether it's on a pole in front of men who want to put cash in your panties, or at the ballet, dancing has always been an excellent exercise.

Snowboarding. 25 mph down a mountain of snow. COOL, or..COLD. Anyway millions find it Fun.

Dig a hole. Get a shovel and dig a hole. Find out what is down there. Maybe you can find Jimmy Hoffa or the Buried Pirate Treasure.

Gold panning. This is a VERY good abdominal and back strengthening exercise AND it just might pay off..in GOLD.

Tree Climbing. You had fun as a kid! Why stop now?

Stir up a hornets nest and see if you can outrun them.

Lumberjacking. YES, very fun for some and VERY physically demanding.

Fly Fishing. No grandpa, you can't just throw your line in and sleep. You need waders and a river to walk up and down.

Military Combat. I hear its hard work killing bad guys.

Peace Marching. I hear its hard work protesting the killing of bad guys.

Ocean Piracy with old sailing vessel. Exhaustive, but scurvy shouldn't be a problem anymore! Just watch out for those Hole Diggin' Bastards, they'll plunder yer' treasure.

Gardening. Plant some Fruits and Veggies and eat them when you get hungry!

Roofing. Use a ladder and Hump them bundles up onto the roof, on your shoulder, one at a time. OH YEAH BUDDY, only the STRONG!

Clean your gutters. Keeps you from having to do Roofing!

Bee Keeping. So you HAVE hornets to run from!

Carpentry. YES, this is what Jesus did. why not you?

The primary thing that you need to overcome if you abhor exercise is your emotional consideration of the action. FIND SOMETHING physical YOU LOVE to do. Find something THAT WILL actually IMPACT YOU.

-No Grandma, knitting isn't going to cut it, nor is playing video games for twelve hours.-

When you think about the exercise you are going to choose, think about your HEART. That's right. Both of them! The emotional one that's all Hurt from breaking up with your Lover and the one made of blood, muscle, tissue, tendon and sinew.

Blood feeds your emotions. Your emotions feed purpose and passion to your actions. Keep your 'Heart' happy.

So how easy is this?

<u>To Exercise; Always follow your HEART!</u>

Can you do that?

Resolve to encourage your HEART HEALTH through HAPPINESS and UTILIZATION!

Link: Your 'Heart' is the core of you. It is the motivational foundation of purpose and it is the physical foundation of ability.

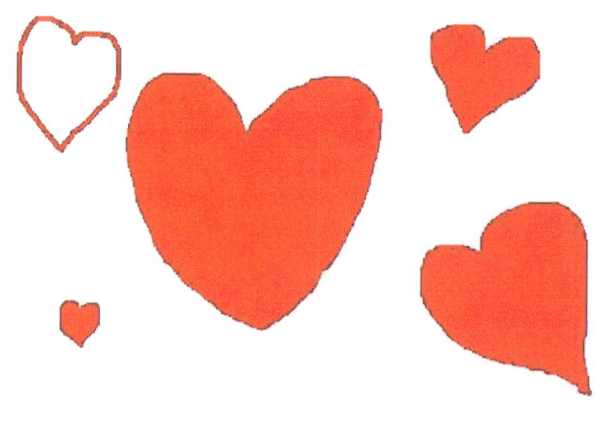

WAIT UNTIL YOU ARE HUNGRY to eat food.

Wait and regulate the Weight. Here's what you are going to do Buck; YOU ARE GOING TO LET GO OF CONTROL. You are going to give control of your food intake Times to your INTERNAL CLOCK and REMOVE power from the WALL CLOCK over YOUR dietary needs. Yes, these are YOUR **_NEEDS_**. This game is the game of SURVIVAL, don't believe anything less and take it SERIOUSLY! PUT YOURSELF FIRST.

That is survival's NUMBER ONE rule.

The boss says, "Lunch is at noon until 1:00". YOU are hungry at 1:45pm. <u>EAT at 1:45pm</u>. If needed explain the situation to your employer. If he or she is inflexible and cannot consider your health as a priority, consider a new job. END any relationship that is detrimental to your health and overall well being. YOUR UNHAPPY DEATH does not help you or your employer either!

Link: Happy Employees are More Productive.

Wait on eating until you feel ACTUAL Hunger. Not gas pain, not heart burn, and not thirst. HUNGER. And while you are waiting to be hungry, drink WATER. Many times stomach sensations are associated as hunger when they are not. Be aware of this, and, KEEP HYDRATED.

Water, WaTeR, WATer, waTER, wATer, WATER, WatER, WAteR, water.! DRINK IT.

You don't need to be Obsessive and measure your quantity down to the sub-molecular level. Just drink it if you feel like ingesting something when not sensing hunger. Do this INSTEAD OF EATING WHEN YOU ARE NOT HUNGRY. Drink lots of water.

Cold pure water. Tepid filtered water. Hot steamy water. Clean refreshing water. Natural Mineral water.

DRINK ENOUGH WATER. Not tea. Not coffee. NOT SODA POP. WATER.

A feeling of a need to ingest can come from many sources. Drinking water during these times will help your biological self assess <u>your</u> actual needs more effectively. When hunger does strike, your craving for a food will help you identify and fulfill your dietary and sustenance needs better, without guessing and without a nutrition book.

Drinking Water regularly will greatly enhance natural metabolic balances. Water is THE BENCHMARK of life on earth. *It is* the master comparison for Chemical regulatory functions.

Link: Alcoholism, GABA, and Sunflower seeds.

Waiting to eat actually has a surprise benefit. Food tastes Dramatically Better. Take Advantage of this FREE taste enhancement and enjoy food MORE! It's literally surprising. Those of you reading this are likely food lovers to some degree or another, why not ENJOY FOOD AGAIN? Quantity will never make it taste this good. Hunger is your friend...to a point.

"But when I'm hungry, what do I eat?"

Food Do's and Don'ts are very Relative to, and Chemically driven by, internal needs. Cravings, for example, are a communication to you of something needed biologically. If you are reading this, YOU ARE LIKELY CRAVING THE WRONG FOODS. This is an attempt of your biology to make sense of what is going on and correct chemical imbalances with the food tools provided.

You will **_NEED_** to follow a better diet. Here are some suggestions:

Do not eat High Fructose Corn Syrup.

Do not eat Partially Hydrogenated oils.

Do not eat monosodium glutamate.

Do not eat Artificial Sweeteners Ever Again!

Un-healthy chemical agents do horrible things to you. Frankly, I suggest you DO NOT EAT ARTIFICIAL ANYTHING! You MUST re-establish your natural HISTORICAL food basis. ***PERIOD***. DO THIS, or you will fail. I won't sugar coat it, only the BRUTAL TRUTH can help you now. Please do it for yourself.

The word here for you to know is CONFUSION. Ever heard of 'tricking your brain' in those weight loss books? Well, you are now FAT because it was TRICKED. Wouldn't a wise individual stop NOW with the tricks? Biological confusion is caused by compounds and agents which seem like something they are not. 'Sweet' that isn't a sugar is an example. Biology knows what you know by 'feel'. Feelings are gained through the association of your five senses and memory reflection. Memory is carried all the way into, and from, the levels of base genetic instinct. THAT IS WHAT INSTINCT IS; MEMORIES. Your internal biology does not run on mathematics.

REPEAT, BIOLOGY DOES NOT RUN ON MATHEMATICS. It never has and it never will. Biology is not based upon math. Doubtful of that? Simply look at the plants and animals of the world.

There aren't too many algebra equations and calculus tests being attempted by Turnips and Barracudas now are there? If you feel like a HOT DOG is meat, yet it is PACKED WITH HIGH FRUCTOSE CORN SYRUP, your biologic reacts in a manner consistent with meat.

Confusion can occur inside the Reptilian Brain: "What the Fuck!? What the hell is this sticky goo? Where did it come from? Why is it in the blood!? I Don't know what to do with it! I Thought meat was coming?? I guess its meat too? ...Oh Crap, why are the Kidneys Shutting down!? OH SHIT, THE HEART STOPPED!" Said the Basal Ganglia to itself as it tried to absorb HIGH FRUCTOSE CORN SYRUP.

Link: R-complex, limbic system, and the Neo-Cortex.

YOU ARE ENTIRELY affected and imbalanced and FLAT OUT POISONED because YOU HAVE BEEN AMBUSHED BY EVIL.

It Really isn't your fault for being mislead and Confused, But; You must take responsibility to CHANGE and not get bush whacked anymore. Adapt. Evolve. Read Labels and become aware of your associated feelings for what you are eating. Track in your mind where the food you are eating came from. If you cannot track an ingredient in your food to it's natural source, DO NOT EAT it. It may be radioactive POISON for all you know. Limit your allowable processing of foods to a known minimum standard, like grinding and powdering. Even mined sources of nutrients like iron and magnesium are ok. It's the MAD SCIENCE CHEMISTRY corporations put in foods to make them taste better you need to DUMP.

Oh yeah, about THAT FAT AND SUGAR intake. LOWER it.

-Yeah I know butter on your pancakes is good and you can track the ingredients to the Udder of a cow and Cane of a field through their processing. So, a Helpful Reminder: THIS IS a FAT MANAGEMENT manual.-

By the way, Check your Pancake Syrup, It may be 100% High Fructose Corn Syrup.

What the hell is that doing in your hot dogs anyway?

SODA POP SUCKS!

Alcohol does too.

Did I mention Tobacco kills you?

Coffee (caffeine) can cause stress. Did you read the part on stress yet?

SODA POP STILL SUCKS!

Emotion altering Drugs Suck!

Weight Loss Drugs Suck!

Stomach Stapling Sucks!

SODA POP; **_STILL_** SUCKS!

Alcohol lowers inhibition. Are you sure you can resist those Macho Nachos and Cheese Fries FATTY?

WATER KICKS ASS!

Un-sweetened Fruit Juice is ok too.

Other Food and drinks Suck too, you must identify and DO NOT EAT FOOD THAT SUCKS. Or Drink it either!

*Un-healthy food agents will change as biology changes. Evolution can eventually allow you to eat these foods without harm. But right now you are fat. Allow your list of unhealthy foods to change, just as you will change. Adapt. Evolve. Survive. Thrive.

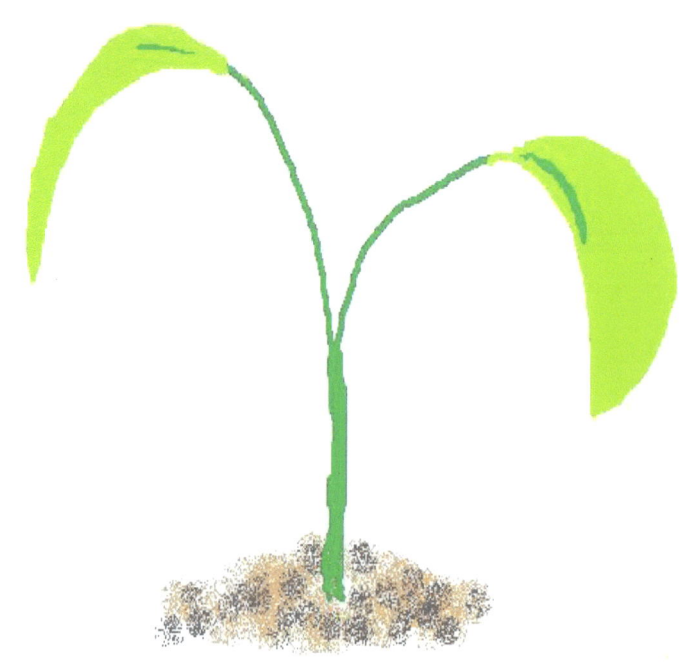

EAT FOOD When You Are Hungry.

At the first sign of actual hunger, **_EAT SOMETHING SLOWLY._** DO NOT STARVE. Starvation triggers fat storage, muscle loss and sedentary lifestyles. Starving makes you feel weak, tired and depressed in an attempt to lower physical energy expenditure. This is an effort to prolong life through conservation of energy. This KEY emotional process goes right along with it's opposite in the biologic of food.

'If there is no Hurry, there is no scarcity and therefore I do not have to store fat'.

If your body doesn't have to do something, it can now expend resources on other tasks, like muscle building and hair growth. As a matter of logical processes, your anatomical system will always do this in order to manage resources effectively and efficiently. It's simple survival prioritization. Confusion is the killer of biologic. Food is one of four top biological priorities. Make food and nutrition a top priority in your lifestyle too.

Your 'Body' trusts your Emotional state of being. This is HOW determination of what to do with food, water, medicines and everything you ingest are made. In fact, biological chemical basis is the only way your body communicates within itself regarding nutritional resource. If your chemistry is off, so are all of the communications.

For example: Tasting high sugar intake communicates to your biology a need for insulin secretion.

Yes. It's that simple.

It is not magic to understand that the only input brains receive come from their sensory organs. There is no other possible mechanical means for your biology to 'know' what you are eating.

-Unless, of course, you are psychic. But if you are, why did you buy this manual? You could have known its contents through Osmosis, or, simply stolen information from the mind of another who has no obesity problem.-

Link: The Blood Brain Barrier.

If you feel 'nervous' or 'hurried' in association with food, Fat storage will result. REMEMBER THIS, KNOW THIS, READ IT FIVE TIMES and THEN do that Religious Chanting thing where you bob your head while reciting it over and over again!

Think about Ancient times, Starvation, and the COMPETITION for food. "I have to eat fast" is an example of this thought. Wouldn't feeling a sense of urgency accompany starving people in their quest to encounter a source of food? These features of your biologic are constructs of BILLIONS OF YEARS OF EXPERIENCE. Trust their reactions and CHANGE your FEELINGS!

WHAT IS THE ACTUAL FOOD SITUATION YOU ARE IN?

SLOWLY! Quit choking it down! Gorging is a behavior Learned as a Tactic in the competition for food and is a BLESSING during Lean times and starvation. Don't be ANGRY at yourself anymore. You NEEDED to eat fast to avoid scavengers, predators and competition in your own tribe. . It happens. It happened to you at some point in your existence too, a lot of times. Don't be ashamed of this behavior; just learn how and WHERE it is a valued ASSET.

Link: Hyena's and lions steal each other's prey.

Eating Slowly Allows you to STOP EATING when you are NO LONGER HUNGRY. By doing so, you allow the proper functioning of your systems to take back charge and Balance your food budgeting based upon the real world and not some hallucination of fear or need. GET REAL about this, I mean REALLY REAL.

MONEY IS NOT FOOD. They are not the same, though, bankers and governments love it when you feel that way. Take a Moment and look around you, at the physical survival situation. NO HYPE. BASE YOUR FOOD MOOD ON THE ACTUAL PHYSICAL VOLUME OF FOOD AVAILABLE TO EAT. Do not put any Money into your evaluation at all! When you are doing your evaluation of resource, ask yourself; "WHAT WOULD YOU ACTUALLY DO IF YOU WERE STARVING?" NOW, look at the resources available to you. That is how you need to EVALUATE FOOD FEELINGS. Are you Starving to death? Would you steal food to eat? I WOULD! How EASY is it to get food? How easy is it REALLY? STOP and take a look at your situation. STOP starving yourself! NEVER EVER EVER STARVE yourself because of money or other stupid reasons again. NEVER EVER AGAIN.

EVER.

Link: Agriculture,   Farming   and Ranching.

Fortunately for you, someone is letting you know you must do a little more than just physically force yourself to slow down eating, you must EMOTIONALLY slow down and ENJOY YOUR MEALS AGAIN. That sense of 'hurry up' and, 'I don't have time for this' needs to go away. This is essential to modifying your fat storing systems. This is how your biological systems monitor and adjust to a changing environment and where you will work to adjust your behaviors for that changing environment too. If people hurry you while eating, tell them to leave. Turn off your phone while eating. And of course, RELAX and take your time. Do not let the Problems of others in Planning and ambition ruin your life anymore. If they 'Urgently need you', let them urgently need you. MAKE THEM WAIT for you to finish. Don't burden yourself further with their emotional stresses. Just drop them, their stress is not that important. It will make them appreciate you more too.

Link: Food is one of four primary resources all animals on earth compete for.

NUTRITION. You saw the Don't list. The do's are much more substantial. Lean meats, raw vegetables and fruits, un-processed foods as much as you can to re-establish your FOUNDATION. Your Foundation is close to the SAME AS it was when you were a HAIRY APE.

-Sorry Religion-

...Anyway Eat Raw Fruits and Vegetables, Whole unprocessed grains, lean meats and eggs and WILD GAME (if you can shoot or buy it). Squirrel is a VERY LOW FAT FOOD. When thinking about your food foundation, consider your historical base and STICK TO IT. This isn't Quantum Theory is it? Start at the level of fire and work from there. Ancient Human-like mammals learned to cook meat. Cooking meat seems to have worked out quite well. Stick to your foundation for a while. Keep things as natural as possible. Eat healthy Foods you LOVE and keep that HEART happy! You will begin to FEEL GREAT. Keep going until you PLATEAU with feeling great. You have reached plateau when this new feeling becomes your NORMAL State of feeling.

Incorporate a <u>QUALITY</u> multi Vitamin if necessary. You MUST Say no to supplements that CAUSE purposeful METABOLIC CHANGE during your period of foundation establishment and plateau. If not, your foundation will be chemically fouled, and therefore, an un-reliable Benchmark from which to judge YOUR actual dietary needs.

Instead of manufacturing a new set of food principles, use the old ones already biologically understood from a million years ago. Your Biological system NEEDS reliable benchmarks to function properly. From Those root chemical bases, you CAN incorporate modern foods. It's your choice which foods to experiment with in the modern world. Some of them can be ok. Afterall, adapting to new food sources is just as important as adapting to anything else.

-Nancy Reagan Said no to drugs, please say no to stimulants and mood enhancers in the form of huge dose vitamins and energy drinks/pills. Do it for your own good. They belong on the SUCK list. You DO NOT want to CONFUSE your NEWLY RECREATED FOOD FEELING BASE, That'd really be bad.-

Once you have hit plateau for a while and chemically stabilize, this new base will be your new food evaluating benchmark. This is how you will now evaluate other foods to incorporate into your diet. If you eat food and you feel like shit, PUT WHATEVER FOOD IT IS WITH WHAT IT FEELS LIKE, IN THE TOILET, and not by eating it first either! Or bury it in the back yard like a cat does, Maybe bag it up with your dog's leavings on his walk and trash it. THAT is where SHIT belongs.

*Diabetics and those of you out there who are in Very Bad Health condition, A Nutritionist and Doctor's Advice is strongly recommended before any radical altering of your diet.

**Sometimes we are faced with decisions in life. Please eat doughnuts, raw lard, High Fructose Corn Syrup, practice cannibalism or whatever else you have to in order to survive starvation and famines. SHIT food is better than no food.

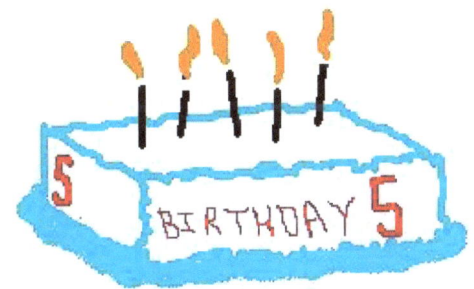

After you have re-established a natural norm, do not eat food that you find makes you Feel Bad. SOME FOODS are designed to make you feel extra good and then CRASH you down. This is a marketing ploy to sell more of the food that made you feel outstanding just a few minutes previously. It's true. You can find out using YOUR NEW FOOD BASE.

-Experiment with known shit foods if you like to feel like crap once in a while and find out for yourself which food and drinks you think suck.-

Was all of that too hard to understand?

If so I could write it in crayons for you.

Link: 'SUPERSIZE ME'. A movie by Morgan Spurlock.

Food feelings and habits are inherited during your formative years with your parents, teachers and family members. Even the dog was an impact on your childhood psychology. T.V. was not a good parent and likely, you have poor habits from others around you, especially people and information sources which were TRUSTED and FED YOU. You may need to learn meditation techniques, therapeutic systems and have a counselor help you to access this area of your mind. RELEARN what you were taught as a child. Aim for the point of origin of the bad habit. In FACT this whole manual is BASED upon this. Treat yourself with respect and remember that as a child, reality was DIFFERENT than it is now. Get in touch with THAT reality, and, make adjustments in that mind frame. BE ABSOLUTELY HONEST with yourself. DO NOT lie to yourself, even to protect your own feelings. It will cause more HARM.

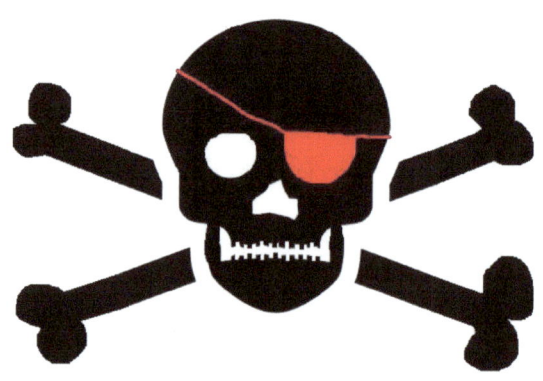

Lying will only cause you MORE pain. Your Pants may end up on fire too!

Link: Hypnotic Regression Therapy and Affirmation of Truth.

RELAX and Adapt.

THAT IS A DIRECT ORDER SOLDIER! You must relax. Stress factors are directly related to your eating habits and Fat Storage on your body. LEARN TO RELAX. This is necessary to begin managing your Fat and the key to engineering a better total self. Rest and relaxation is one of the essentials to successful muscle building, athletic training, and overall health. You need to sleep and relax.

Link: Sleep Apnea.

Stress associated with food intake directly affects metabolism in the following manner:

It causes FAT STORAGE and MUSCLE LOSS.

These actions are formed through biological reasoning:

'If I am stressing over food, there must be a scarcity, therefore I must lower my food requirements (SEDENTARY TACTICS and MUSCLE LOSS) and increase my food storage (FAT GAIN) in order to survive through this scarcity'.

This is Biologic. Your Biologic may have angered you. STOP RIGHT NOW BEING ANGRY AT YOURSELF, it will not serve you to hate yourself. It IS logical when you think about it. How many times have you survived through famines, droughts, and other resource scarcities over the billions of years you have existed on earth? This life is not your first and you KNOW that. Instead of getting mad, USE your survival and instinct system and modify your behavior and feelings accordingly. This isn't the first time you have had to ADAPT to a situation is it? Are you going to let it be your LAST?

Increasing your activity will change your biological functioning to the other side of the reasoning scale: 'Due to food being difficult to capture and ingest, I must expend and metabolize fat, increase muscle mass, and release strengthening hormones to ACQUIRE more food and survive through this scarcity.'

Does that make sense to you? It should.

A lighter, more efficient, physical make up requires less effort to move around and requires less energy to support. This is the opposite but equally important procedural process within the biological mind calculated sub consciously throughout your everyday life and through every famine you have survived thus far. Again, it is based upon your emotional assessment. It is a METHODICAL CALCULATION. This is where the balance is struck between SEDENTARY OR ACTIVE life styling and this is where your emotional work needs active focus to successfully achieve MANAGING YOUR FAT.

If you have EMOTIONAL PROBLEMS like DEPRESSION, STOP RIGHT HERE. Mark the page. Pick up the phone and dial the doctor or an ambulance and GET YOUR BUTT SOME MEDICAL ATTENTION NOW!

This manual cannot help you unless you are ABLE to help yourself. Pay the Fees, find help from the county health agency, go to the emergency room, call a suicide hotline. DO WHATEVER YOU HAVE TO DO and THROW FEAR ASIDE. Fear of taking ACTION due to embarrassment or Prideful Delusions will never make your problem go away. If you do not know what to do, JUST TRY SOMETHING. Ask a stranger on the street if you can't figure anything else out.

-HELL, Stand in traffic and piss yourself until the police take notice. Get the help you need once you are in jail.-

Take your situation SERIOUSLY. KNOW THAT YOUR LIFE IS ON THE LINE HERE PAL!

The absolute KEY TO EVERYTHING is YOUR BRAIN. It CONTROLS ALL OF YOUR ACTIONS ABSOLUTELY!

Momma says; "If the Brain ain't healthy, *ain't- NOTHIN'- Else- gonna'- Be- Healthy- either!"*

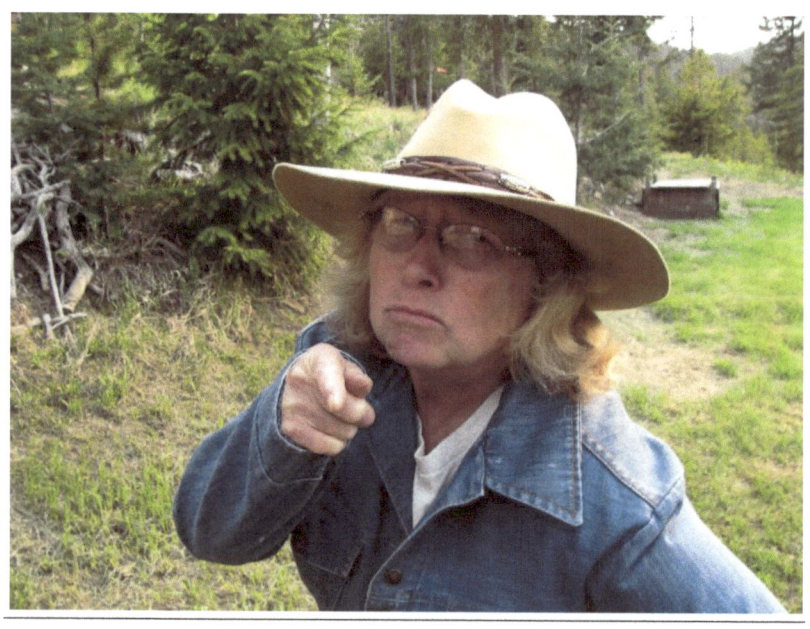

Do not be ashamed if you have a mental illness of some type, just get it treated. You would take Antibiotics if you caught Chlamydia wouldn't you?

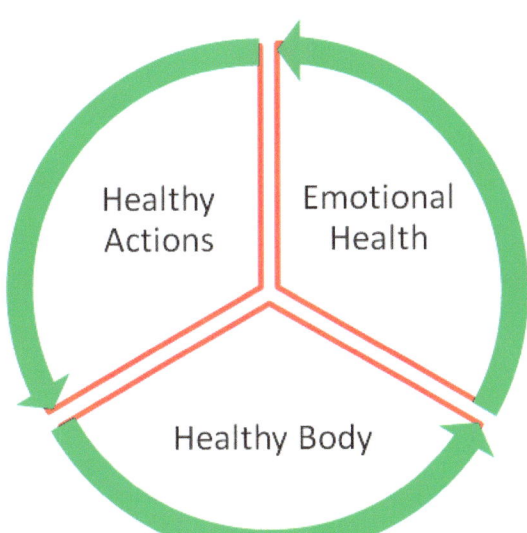

Link: Depression is a problem of the emotional Heart. Humans will shy away from emotionally depressed people because feelings are shared just like the warmth of a fire.

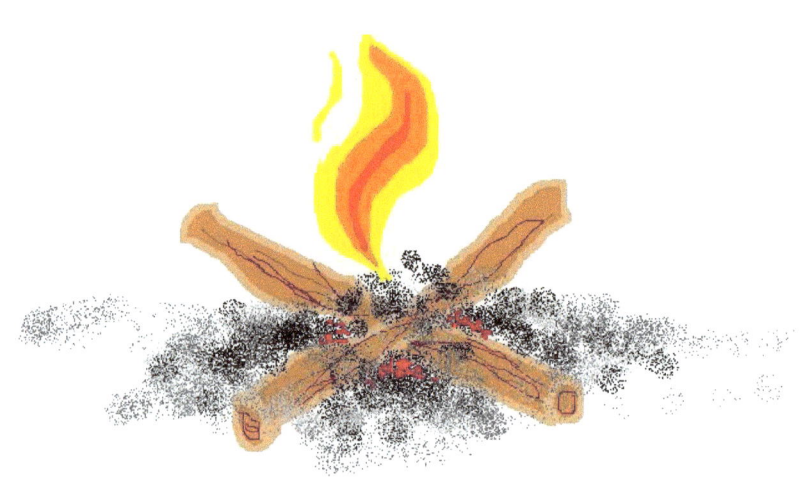

*A note on bodybuilding and athletic physiques;

Bodybuilders and athletes have Heart. They are doing what they do because they LOVE what they do! They have a passion for improving themselves. Do not compare yourself to these people unless you LOVE to compete in sport. You can dishearten your RESOLVE and fail yourself. Do not place these expectations on yourself unless you LOVE ATHLETIC PARTICIPATION. This goes for any comparison you are making. Keep your expectations reasonable and/or open. These people's bodies have conformed to the demands of the sport they compete within. That's all there is to it!

You will not likely SUCCEED at having an ATHLETIC PHYSIQUE without first loving the associated sport that demands that physique.

Almost all serious professional athletes spend THOUSAND if not MILLIONS of dollars and HUNDREDS OF HOURS yearly on personal training. That's a whole lot of time they could have been gold panning and diggin' up pirate treasure!

-Why limit the OUTCOME of your endeavor to the limits imposed by someone else's actions or life? Do the best you can and find your POTENTIAL, Maybe you have hidden mutant powers or something you just need to unleash! -

So, quit hurting yourself right now. Start becoming the best YOU can be. You might find it surprising later how many people become JEALOUS of how awesome YOU are.

Repeat Steps 2 through 5 for the rest of your life.

Repeating the steps it takes for the remainder of your life will ELIMINATE the YOYO Problem completely. The problem with dieting is the feeling of COMPLETION and success. The feeling of success is great, but, can allow feelings of justification for, and a return to; poor HABITS. The feeling of success is the root cause of the yoyo effect in dieting. Stop believing you are finished with your 'diet'. A diet is what you eat, not a game, a competition, or a burden. You must re-associate diet with food and eliminate the emotional relationship of 'dieting' to obesity.

You feel like an unsuccessful loser as a FATTY, LOSING UN-HEALTHY FAT CREATES A FEELING OF ACCOMPLISHMENT AND SELF WORTH.

Many times this fundamental feeling of self worth becomes so needed, in this idealistic beauty obsessive world, the brain causes you to gain fat, and lose it again, just to create that feeling of self worth missing in your life! STOP! You MUST find a new way to experience those delightful feelings and ACCOMPLISH a HAPPIER YOU.

How about completing a marathon if you enjoy running? Accomplish THOSE kinds of goals and enjoy a feeling of achievement! Foot races are a perfect example of a true start and finish exercise, and are supported by a proper food foundation. Leave DIETING behind you now. "Dieting" IS NOT the CORRECT mindset for maintaining a proper body fat percentage nor will it help you in your quest to survive or MAINTAIN SELF ESTEEM.

When you are on a prescribed and/or regimented diet, there is a feeling of a start and finish. A timeline is presented through your weight loss goals. Most only adhere to the "diet" attempting to attain those goals. There is no Beginning, nor is there an end to your need to SURVIVE. Survival is the proper mindset to establish your dietary traditions and habits from. SURVIVAL IS YOUR ONLY TRUE GOAL NOW! YOU MUST FOLLOW THROUGH! CONTINUE to adapt and better yourself.

Humans tend to survive better and longer when they feel as if they have something to LIVE for. Find that something, EXERCISE with that purpose. DETERMINATION was needed during your days as a Neanderthal. It's still needed now.

-Maybe an obsessive compulsive disorder would be a good thing when it comes to survival? Maybe that's how you use OBSESSION and COMPULSION in a fundamentally positive manner. -

So, now that you have the dutiful Information you need, let's simplify this to a sentence or three:

Have fun doing something energetic. As hunger drifts in, make an engaged food decision somewhere and have a leisurely meal. Go home and sleep on your nice, cozy, pillow top bed as drowsiness beckons you to the world of Dreams and Dreamers.

Think you can handle this?

If not, maybe someone needs to beat you with a stick.

Some people are *into* that sort of thing.

Maybe you can find a Fat Management buddy who likes that kind of 'Exercise'.

www.ingramcontent.com/pod-product-compliance
Lightning Source LLC
Chambersburg PA
CBHW050817290526
45792CB00001B/160